D0436359

DESTINATION

SIMPLE

Brooke McAlary produces and hosts The Slow Home, an iTunes #1 Health podcast. Brooke blogs about decluttering and slow living at slowyourhome.com

DESTINATION

SIMPLE

**EVERYDAY RITUALS
FOR A SLOWER LIFE**

BROOKE MCALARY

ANIMA

First published in Australia in 2017 by Nero,
an imprint of Schwartz Publishing Pty Ltd

First published in the UK by Anima,
an imprint of Head of Zeus Ltd, in 2017

9 7 5 3 1 2 4 6 8

A catalogue record for this book is available
from the British Library

ISBN (HB): 9781786694416
ISBN (E): 9781786694409

Printed and bound in Germany by CPI Books GmbH

Cover design by Jen Clark Design
Text design and typesetting by Tristan Main
Cover image: Giada Canu, Stocksy

Head of Zeus Ltd
First Floor East
5–8 Hardwick Street
London EC1R 4RG

WWW.HEADOFZEUS.COM

To my family: You've been the making of
me. I love you all to the moon and back.

To everyone who has read
or listened to Slow Your Home over the
past few years: thank you.

Hi, I'm Brooke! I'm a thirty-something recovering burnout living in the Blue Mountains, just outside Sydney, Australia, with my wonderful family, dog, chickens and ever-evolving garden. I'm a writer, an inappropriate laugher and an advocate for the best things in life – siestas, time spent outside, travel and the lost art of doing nothing. I'm also someone who, after a period of darkness, ill-health and upheaval, decided to simplify my life and the life of my family.

Step by step. Piece by piece. Day by day.

And largely, I've been successful.

I've decluttered our family home of thousands of unwanted items and organised it to a point that works for us. I feel physically lighter and am more content, and am prone to unexpected bursts of happiness. I also dance while sweeping, sing while driving and actually enjoy playing with my kids. I'm a changed person and my family is a changed family, all because we adopted the idea of living more simply.

I hope you'll join me . . .

/

Contents

We're so caught up in trying to do everything, experience all the essential things, not miss out on anything important ...

We can't read all the good books, watch all the good films, go to all the best cities in the world, try all the best restaurants, meet all the great people ... Life is better when we don't try to do everything.

Learn to enjoy the slice of life you experience, and life turns out to be wonderful.

LEO BABAUTA

Introduction

In the modern world we live life in the fast lane. We race to keep up with the Joneses. We are overworked, overconnected and overstressed, and we compete over how busy, important and sleep-deprived we are. But we don't have to.

An ever-growing number of people are opting out of a life lived at 110%. They are choosing to slow down, simplify, say no and focus on the things that are truly important. I'm one of them, and deciding to live a slower, simpler life has been hands down one of the best decisions I've ever made, for both my own wellbeing and that of my family.

Before I chose to slow down and simplify, I was an overwhelmed, overcommitted wreck. I was so stressed I could barely function. I realised later that I had lived my entire adult life in a state of low-grade panic. There was no downtime, no peace, no space, no margin, no buffer – and nothing remotely close to slow.

I spent my days trying to do dozens of things at once and becoming increasingly frustrated that I was doing none of those things well. I wasn't present as a parent, partner, friend, business owner, daughter or sister. I felt fractured but completely incapable of taking my foot off the accelerator. If I slowed down, wouldn't all the delicate balls I had in the air smash on the floor, leaving me with nothing to show for any of it? Truth be told, I was terrified.

We know there's more to life than constant rush, excess stuff, endless notifications, breakfast in the car and mindless TV at the end of the day. We catch occasional glimpses of that something more – downtime, uncluttered headspace, wandering, spontaneity, a moment spent lingering in the sunshine – but more often than not is covered in a thick layer of 'shoulds', 'must haves', 'to dos' and 'need-to-be-seens'. We're terrified of what we'll discover if we let ourselves slow down, if we take the time to question our decisions, if we open ourselves up to some self-awareness.

This little book is a hard-won collection of ideas that worked for me as I learnt to simplify my mind, my days and my home. I hope they will help you simplify your life one small step at a time and start finding tiny pockets of space for quiet, peace, calm and happiness. It doesn't need to be terrifying and it doesn't need to feel out of reach. You can start creating a slower, simpler life today.

For most people, the journey towards simplicity starts with decluttering their stuff: clearing out wardrobes, or sorting through books, photos and decades of sentimental items. As they look around their home in frustration, they declare,

'That's it! I'm buying fewer shoes/clothes/tennis racquets/toys/books/CDs. I'm sick of clearing this stuff out!' But fast-forward twelve months and you'll find many of them are back at it, grumbling about how they would prefer to be watching TV, relaxing, drinking a beer or playing with their kids. Instead, they're clearing out the garage again.

In this little book I'll show you that instead of trying – and repeatedly failing – to get the physical clutter sorted, you need to first free up a little space in your daily life.

If you change the flow of your days – making them a little simpler, lighter and easier – the physical decluttering will follow.

This is not a book to help you organise your home. It's not about creating the perfect filing system or establishing a routine of regular clutter-busting. It won't tell you the 'right' way to organise your pantry or simplify your wardrobe. Instead, it will show you that by being intentional with your daily actions you can create the simpler, happier life you want. And you can do this by harnessing the power of rituals and rhythms.

USING THIS BOOK

This is a small book.

It's intentionally brief, because I know you're busy and frustrated with how hectic life is. That's why you've picked this book up – you're looking for ways to reduce that busy-ness and feeling of being overwhelmed. The good news is, this book offers seven solutions.

Choosing to adopt all seven of these rituals and rhythms is the easiest, most successful way to create a simpler, slower life. However, even incorporating just one of these into your daily life will make a positive impact and might give you momentum to make further changes.

I suggest you read the entire book first. Many of the rhythms and rituals flow into each other, and while it may sound like a lot of work in the beginning, applying all of them together will save you a great deal of time and effort.

This book doesn't prescribe exact actions. It won't tell you how to change your life – not exactly.

It will, however, arm you with a framework to help you change your own life for the better.

A PEP TALK BEFORE WE BEGIN...

Life is busy. You don't have time to try anything new. I hear you. I understand. And I used to think the very same thing. But the truth is, if you're telling me (and yourself) that you don't have time, then you really do need this book.

The reality of making change in your life is that:

it takes *effort*

it takes *time*

it takes *energy*.

But the payoff can be enormous: a simpler, happier life that doesn't require endless readjustment and constant planning.

That's the beauty of rhythms and rituals. Once established, they become part of your daily life. You don't need to schedule them, just like you don't schedule brushing your teeth or going to bed. Everything just flows.

So if you find yourself feeling overwhelmed at the work involved in some of the exercises in this book, focus on what you stand to gain.

And remember: every journey starts with one small step.

PART ONE

RITUALS

A ritual is a formal, ceremonial task that is undertaken regularly. The term often has religious connotations. Rituals have weight and significance, and people approach them with a measure of importance.

In this book, I'm taking that idea of a 'ritual' and applying it to everyday life. I'm asking you to give weight and significance to some of the things you do on a daily basis. Doing this elevates these tasks beyond the mundane and helps you to truly appreciate and pay attention to what it is you're doing.

You will be surprised how simple the tasks in this section are. There's no need for complicated productivity methods or in-depth activity audits. This book is about simple ideas for a simpler life. Complex time management systems are not my style. Simple ideas to help you do less while living more? That's what we're aiming for.

When tea becomes ritual, it takes its place at the heart of our ability to see greatness in small things. Where is beauty to be found? In great things that, like everything else, are doomed to die, or in small things that aspire to nothing, yet know how to set a jewel of infinity in a single moment?

MURIEL BARBERY

1

Single-tasking

Do you multi-task? Often find yourself doing two or more things at once?

Of course you do – everyone does.

- You plan dinner while making breakfast.

- You write your presentation while in another meeting.

- You hang the washing while you talk to your kids.

- You listen to an audiobook while you exercise.

- You talk on the phone while stacking the dishwasher.

It's what you're supposed to do, right?

You multi-task because you're clever. Because you're efficient. You're making the most of your time. You're getting things sorted.

Yes, in some instances, multi-tasking can be a positive thing, a way to get tasks done quickly and efficiently, freeing us to spend time on the things we really want to be doing.

But what about the other side of the coin?

- Do you feel exhausted?

- Like you're not doing anything well?

- Like you're being torn in too many directions?

Despite what your overwhelmed, overworked, overcommitted brain may be telling you, you don't need to do more.

You need to **single-task**.

Focus on just one thing at a time.

Not only is single-tasking the opposite of multi-tasking (obviously), it's also a chance to practise complete mindfulness on the task at hand.

Single-tasking is the antidote to modern life, where we are taught that to be effective, productive and worthwhile, we must multi-task.

IT'S NOT ABOUT DOING LESS

As enticing as it sounds, focusing only on the task at hand all day, every day is impractical.

Instead, the ritual of single-tasking involves:

- choosing one task you regularly do during your day

- focusing solely on that task

- immersing yourself wholly and completely in experiencing it.

It helps you find the simple beauty and everyday joy in mindfully completing one task.

Practising this ritual of mindfulness brings you completely into the present moment. It teaches you how to be grateful for even the most mundane of tasks and opens your mind to the beauty of doing one thing wholeheartedly.

It might not be possible to single-task for your whole life – or even a whole day. But practising single-tasking once a day is entirely achievable. And it adds no time, as you choose a task you already do. Now this task serves an extra purpose: it's a chance to clear the mental clutter – even for a moment.

The best way to make single-tasking worthwhile is to focus on the right things at the right time – to discern the difference between distractions and purpose.

JOSHUA BECKER

Single-tasking

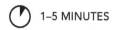 1–5 MINUTES

Five minutes is all you need for this exercise. Even one minute will do. One minute of beautiful, meditative quiet in a day otherwise filled with the urgent need to be productive, get things done, prove your value.

1. PICK ONE TASK

Choose an everyday task, such as brushing your teeth, making the bed, hanging out the laundry or washing up after dinner. When the time comes to do that task, devote yourself to it completely.

2. SOAK UP EVERY DETAIL

Immerse yourself in your senses. Let this task be the one thing you are thinking about, the sole purpose of this moment.

Are you hanging out the laundry? Instead of planning dinner or thinking about tomorrow's meeting or what you will do when the kids wake from their nap, focus on:

- the fresh scent of the wet, clean clothes

- the coolness of the damp fabric in your hands

- the snap of the pegs on the line

- the way the sunlight hits the linen.

Appreciate that you're making time to do this simple task so your family will have clean clothes.

Perhaps you're making a cup of tea:

- Think about the water heating up in the kettle.

- As you pour the water into the cup, concentrate on the comforting sound it makes.

- Watch the tea leaves stain the water, changing it from transparent to light to dark.

- If you add milk, watch it combine with the water, changing its colour.

- If you add sugar, listen to the clink of your spoon on the sides of the cup as you stir.

- Notice how the steam rises delicately.

3. WHEN YOU'RE DONE . . .

Take a deep breath and return to the day.

Get back to keeping balls in the air, kids on swings, food in bellies, phone calls answered – but with a newly created pocket of time and a sense of mindfulness you might not have had otherwise.

WHY MAKE IT A RITUAL?

By making this small ritual of single-tasking part of your everyday life, you are prioritising your wellbeing. You are acknowledging that there is more to life than churning through a to-do list, more than just getting things done. After all, this is why we're on the path to a simpler life, isn't it? So we can experience more of these moments every day. More simple pleasures. More little joys. More mindful intention.

The true secret of happiness
lies in taking a genuine interest in all
the details of daily life.

WILLIAM MORRIS

2

Unplugging

In 1999, Dr Donald Wetmore, a time management expert, noted that the average person at that time received more information on a daily basis than the average person born in 1900 received in a *lifetime*. Given that in the twenty-first century we are constantly connected to our smartphones, wifi and social media, you can safely assume the amount of information we receive daily has skyrocketed even further in the past seventeen years.

And we need a break.

We need time to ourselves. Time to let the noise, stimulus and information subside. Time when we're not trying to cram more in.

Our constantly connected world has many advantages. We can communicate across vast distances, experience incredible places virtually, learn from masters and discover anything imaginable with a few clicks of a mouse button or the swipe of a finger.

But being constantly connected has disadvantages too. We carry our smartphones in our pockets, using them as cameras, calendars, notebooks and alarm clocks. We feel naked without at least one source of connection – an iPad, smartphone, laptop or all three.

We have forgotten how to simply be. How to immerse ourselves in what is in front of us. How to truly engage in face-to-face conversation, personal connections and true downtime. And we are burning out, completely addicted to this digital connection.

We're afraid that if we unplug we will miss out on something.

We're afraid that if we aren't involved in everything, we won't be seen as important, we'll be forgotten.

But the price we pay for this constant level of connection is steep – unless we learn to offset our digital lives with periods of disconnection.

THE POWER OF THE OFF SWITCH

Disconnection from the online world allows us to reconnect fully with the world around us – our kids, our partner, our family, our friends, our work, our environment, our imagination.

THE RITUAL OF UNPLUGGING

This ritual involves taking time every day to unplug from the constantly connected world.

It means unplugging from your laptop, email, smartphone and TV.

Sounds incredibly simple, doesn't it?

But once you start to think about your day and consider how you spend your down time, you might start realising it won't be so easy.

Think about it – how do you like to unwind? A glass of wine at the end of the day? Reading a book? Flicking through a magazine? Spending time in the garden? Wonderful!

What about reading blogs? Or ebooks? Watching TV while you enjoy that glass of wine? Flicking through a digital version of your magazine? Not to mention Facebook? Twitter? Instagram?

These may be ways you like to relax, but you are still connected. The virtual world is still there, pulling you in thirty-two opposite directions at once, tempting you to learn more, see more, know more.

So often we open our smartphone to take a look at something specific, but before we realise what's happened we've spent twenty minutes scrolling through Instagram, checking work emails out of office hours or googling the name of the guy on *The Walking Dead* to see if he's the guy from *Love, Actually* (for the record, he is).

It's so easy to act passively online …
checking email isn't necessarily responding
or taking action, but we do it anyway.

COURTNEY CARVER

EXERCISE

Unplugging

 15–30 MINUTES

1. IDENTIFY A TIME

Look at your daily schedule and find a block of 15–30 minutes when you can be off the grid. Choose a time of day when you are unlikely to receive urgent phone calls and when your boss won't need you.

2. SCHEDULE IT

Once you've nominated a block of time – preferably the same time each day – schedule it in your diary or calendar as your down time.

3. COMMIT TO IT

Set a reminder alarm on your computer and phone. Set it to sound twice – once five minutes before your unplugging time begins (allowing you to wrap up any tasks before you disconnect) and then again to signal when it's time to unplug. When you hear that second alarm, close your laptop, take your phone out of your pocket and put it away, switch off the TV and find yourself back in the land of the living.

4. ADD A PRE-BED BLOCK

Try adding a second block of unplugged time to your pre-bed routine.

There's increasing research suggesting that evening screen-time or exposure to blue light (from your smartphone, laptop, tablet or TV screen) not only impacts our brain's ability to recognise that it's night and therefore time for sleep, but also affects the quality of the sleep we do get.

Removing all technology from the bedroom has been a game-changer in our home, resulting in better quality sleep and calmer, more productive mornings. We don't wake up to our phones and dive into emails, news and social media first thing anymore. As you read on you'll see why starting your mornings without technology will help you to establish more positive rituals in your day.

A NOTE ON REALITY

I understand how difficult it can be to find uninterrupted time during the day. Whether you work nine to five in an office or you're home with the kids, life is busy.

But unplugging is such an important ritual for simplifying your life; I really encourage you to find the time. If that's proving hard, try one of these ideas:

• Break your unplugging time into two blocks of 10–15 minutes.

- Try unplugging on the bus or train on your way to and from work.

- Get up earlier and enjoy the early morning quiet without plugging in to your computer or phone – emails can wait 15 minutes.

- Leave for the gym 15 minutes earlier and find a quiet spot to sit.

- Watch one less television show at night.

- Make a real effort to cut back on social media. How many feeds do you really need to scroll through anyway? Try cutting your social media use in half and spend that time offline instead.

WHAT TO DO INSTEAD?

You could try:

- sitting quietly

- reading

- walking

- playing with your kids

- writing

- talking with your partner

- prayer

- meditation

- yoga

- sipping a coffee outside, watching the sky, hearing the birds.

Whatever you choose to do while you unplug, the important thing is that you connect with the real world, or allow your mind to access a different virtual one – the world of your own imagination.

3

Emptying your mind

Our minds are cluttered. We are overwhelmed with to-do items, commitments, errands and must-remembers.

It's uncomfortable and unproductive to operate at such a high level of stress and tension. From experience I can attest to the fact that leaving this stuff in your head for days and weeks at a time affects other parts of your life.

Do you ever:

- get to bed, begin to relax, only to magically remember everything you were supposed to get done that day?

- find yourself sitting down to watch a movie, only to reach for your smartphone or laptop in order to catch up on the tasks you forgot to do during the day?

- find your mind wandering off at inopportune moments (like in a meeting or during an intimate moment with your partner) to mull over all the things you need to get done?

Thought so. Me too.

Annoying, isn't it? Your brain doesn't seem to appreciate that you're trying to sleep, relax or love. It's still processing information.

The good news? This daily ritual can help.

BRAIN DUMPING

Brain dumping is a mind-mapping or journaling exercise where you simply, well … dump the contents of your brain onto paper.

By doing so, you release your pent-up frustrations, problems, worries and to-dos. Getting it out on paper means it no longer occupies space in your mind, leaving you to think more clearly.

Exactly how you go about this ritual is up to you. Experiment to find what works for your lifestyle and the way you think and process information. Essentially, though, it involves taking 5–10 minutes a day to empty your brain of extraneous information. Just open the floodgates and let it out. Most of what you write will be utter junk. But it's certainly better out than in!

Once it's down on paper, your brain can do its thing without hindrance. It can process the immediate information and deal in the present, rather than being weighed down by thinking about the past and future.

WHAT'S INVOLVED?

You'll need 5–10 minutes for this ritual. But the beauty of it is that you can combine it with your three things ritual (Chapter 4) and your gratitude exercises (Chapter 5) and get three times the benefits at once. Read on and you'll see how.

WHEN IS THE BEST TIME?

It's probably best to do this ritual either first thing in the morning or last thing at night. Usually everyone else is quiet, happy or sleeping at these times, so you won't be interrupted.

But the exact best time for you will depend on your daily flow. You'll get a much better idea about this after working through your morning and evening rhythms (Chapters 6 and 7).

BENEFIT OF MORNINGS

When you're fresh from sleep, you can quickly identify what the day holds, what needs doing and how you're feeling. Brain dumps in the morning help you start positively and begin the day with purpose and a clear mind.

BENEFIT OF EVENINGS

Some people find they sleep better after doing this exercise at night. Issues or grievances they hadn't been paying attention to will find their way to the page and once these are out, they feel physically calmer and more inclined to sleep well. Doing this ritual at night also means you wake up knowing what the next day holds. You've spent the time ordering your thoughts and you can dive into the day without too much planning. Just get moving.

EXERCISE

Emptying your mind

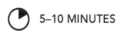 5–10 MINUTES

This is a low-tech ritual. It's about using your hands to empty your mind.

1. FIND A QUIET MOMENT

Five minutes is enough time, but ten is probably better. Regardless of how long you choose, commit to that time.

To begin with, especially, you might find it easiest to set a timer.

2. GRAB A PEN AND PAPER

Pen and paper are underrated these days. The old-school method is infinitely better for this exercise than keyboard and screen or tablet and finger; it allows you to mindmap freely and limits the potential for distractions like email and social media.

3. SIMPLY WRITE

Without thinking too much, write down:

- things you need to remember

- tasks you need to complete

- problems that have been worrying you

- possible solutions

- grocery items you need to buy

- scheduled events

- social occasions coming up

- outfits you want to wear

- chores you need to do

- funny things your kids have said

- anything else you want to capture.

If you find yourself with nothing to write, simply write, 'I have nothing to write. I have nothing to write. I have noth …' I guarantee your brain will offer something up soon enough.

Don't censor yourself; just let it flow. Don't worry about neatness, spelling or grammar.

4. MAP IT OUT

As themes and ideas start to take shape, add arrows, squares and emphasis marks between linked items, or underline or highlight various parts. This helps you to visualise what's happening in your brain and clarify what's essential to pay attention to and, importantly, what can be forgotten.

When your timer goes off, you can stop.

5. COMBINE WITH OTHER RITUALS

One of the reasons I recommend reading through this book completely before beginning the exercises is because so many of the rituals are interlinked. While they will all help you simplify your life on their own, combining them increases the impact and saves you time.

4

Three things

We are drowning in to-do lists.

We've been taught that the longer the list, the more important we are. The more ticks we have on our list, the more efficient, smart, productive or successful we are. At least, that's the thinking.

Do you have items on your to-do list from yesterday? Last week? Last month? Last year?

If something has been on your to-do list for weeks or months, ask yourself: are you ever really going to make time to do it?

Probably not.

That item is just taunting you, reminding you how ineffective, lazy, unproductive and undisciplined you are. Which is not terribly conducive to, you know, getting things done!

BE GONE, LONG TO-DO LISTS!

Long to-do lists do not help to simplify life. They clutter it up. They weigh you down. They make for frustration and anxiety and disappointment and feelings of not being good enough.

So we're doing away with long to-do lists.

Instead, try creating a to-do list of just three items. The three things you need to achieve today.

WHY THREE?

We overcommit ourselves when we write long to-do lists. We know we can't complete the thirty-nine tasks on our list today, yet we still write them down with the expectation they will be done. We set ourselves up to fail before we even begin. However, with three items:

- our goals are achievable – on all but the worst days

- our goals are actionable – the list is not overwhelming

- our goals are simple – you won't lose track of what you're working on.

And you get a victory – three, in fact! You will feel a huge sense of achievement when you complete your to-dos on a regular basis. No more failures.

'BUT THERE ARE MORE THAN THREE THINGS I NEED TO DO DAILY . . .'

Absolutely. The things that are a daily occurrence – making the bed, doing a load of laundry, cooking dinner, dropping kids to school – should be part your daily rhythms, not your to-do list. We will explore those daily tasks in Chapters 6 and 7.

The three things should come from the less frequent, but important 'one-off' tasks that are floating around in your head (which is why I recommend combining this exercise with the brain dump): reports you need to write, phone calls you need to make, appointments, errands.

Each morning, you will nominate the three most important or time-sensitive of these tasks and work to get those done.

You can even create two separate lists – one for work and one for home, to keep you focused in each area throughout the day.

This way you're making it easy for yourself and removing the pressure you put on yourself to do everything in any one given day. The sense of achievement you will feel from actually completing your to-do lists is also incredibly motivating and means you are more likely to continue and achieve even more.

Three things

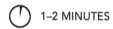 1–2 MINUTES

You can combine this ritual with your brain dump ritual (Chapter 3). Alternatively, you may already know what your three most important tasks are for the day. In that case, start with step two.

1. REVIEW BRAIN DUMP

Once you've finished your brain dump, take a minute to look over what you've written and identify any recurring issues or urgent problems. This is a good opportunity to create two separate lists if needed – one for your home tasks and one for work.

- Is there anything you can do today to improve things?

- Are there any specific tasks that need doing?

- Is there anything on the page that is time-sensitive?

Circle those items.

2. LIST IT OUT

Using pen and paper, list the three most pressing items. These are your top three. Do these before any other tasks.

3. SECONDARY TASKS

You can also list other, less-urgent tasks that need doing – but no more than five or six. Only if you've completed your top three should you move on to the secondary tasks.

4. FOLLOW UP

When you next do the exercise you can move the secondary tasks, as well as any new tasks that need doing, to the following day's list. Simply identify the next three most important items.

I'm all about simplicity and not overcomplicating matters. So, for me, a notebook or paper is ample for my to-do list. You could have one notebook for your home list and one for your work tasks. If you're after a daily planner with a little more structure and more space, there are plenty of excellent daily planners available online.

5

Gratitude

You know those people who always see the glass as half full? Who see the best in people? Who can spot opportunities disguised as disappointment?

They share something in common:

GRATITUDE

Recent studies have shown that those of us who are regularly grateful for the good in our lives are likely to be more physically active, feel more content in our day-to-day lives and suffer fewer health problems.

The key is to regularly spend time being aware of and grateful for the good in our lives. To actively stop taking these everyday blessings for granted. To pause, look around and say, 'Hey, it's OK. My life might not be perfect. And I may not be running marathons / curing cancer / raising kids / travelling / out of debt / achieving whatever other goal I've set, but I am me. And that's pretty great, for these reasons.'

Like anything worthwhile, feeling positive and grateful takes time, effort and patience and – above all – practice. In this section, you'll learn how to integrate the practice of gratitude into your daily life, so that soon it becomes a natural part of every day.

So leave negativity, comparisons and self-doubt at the door – they only get in the way of living the simpler life you want. And become one of those positive-minded people you admire.

EXERCISE

Gratitude

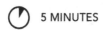 5 MINUTES

1. FIND TIME

Find a small window of time during your day – five minutes is enough. First thing upon waking is perfect, as is last thing before sleep. But any time you can grab a few minutes is great.

You could also combine this exercise with your brain dump and three things rituals. You're spending a few minutes writing anyway – why not work through all three rituals together?

2. WRITE IT DOWN

On a scrap of paper, in a fancy book or on a

chalkboard in the kitchen – wherever suits you – make a list of five things you are grateful for today.

Keep it brief. Don't go overboard – just a few words about each thing is enough. A sentence at the most is all you need to remind yourself of the good things in your life right now. Then reflect on those things, acknowledge them as positive elements in your life, and remind yourself that there are things worth being grateful for in every single day – no matter how bad the day might have been, or what looms in the day ahead.

3. FLIP IT

If you find it difficult to articulate those good things, try flipping your frustrations, anger or resentments. Ask yourself: what about this situation is positive?

- Can't get a moment to yourself? Your kids love you and want to be with you – how beautiful.

- Constantly interrupted at work? People need you or respect your insights – take pride in that.

- Tired of cooking every night? You're providing for your family – there are so many things in that one idea to be grateful for.

One of the most tragic things I know about human nature is that all of us tend to put off living. We are all dreaming of some magical rose garden over the horizon instead of enjoying the roses that are blooming outside our windows today.

DALE CARNEGIE

Summary

Single-tasking (1–5 minutes)

- Choose one task in your day and devote yourself wholly to it.

- Soak up all that this one task entails – the smells, sounds, sights and feel of it.

- Immerse yourself and be completely mindful for that one moment.

Unplugging (15–30 minutes)

- For at least 15 minutes a day, unplug completely: no TV, phones, computer, Kindle, iPad. Nothing.

- Use this time to read, write, play or simply do nothing at all.

- Try adding another chunk of unplugged time before bed and notice the impact it has on your sleep.

Emptying your mind (5–10 minutes)

- Take some time – ideally in the morning or at night – to brain dump. Write out all your worries, distractions, to-dos and thoughts onto the page.

- Underline, circle or connect things as needed to clarify what is on your mind and what actions you need to take.

Three things (1–2 minutes)

- Using your brain dump, choose the three tasks that are most important to complete today.

- Don't move on to any other tasks until these are done.

Gratitude (5 minutes)

- When brain dumping, write down five things you are grateful for in your life. Just a word or two for each is enough.

- If you're struggling to find things to be grateful for, try finding the positives to any perceived negatives.

PART TWO

RHYTHMS

Rhythm. It's the beat of your day. The tempo, the sequence, the order.

You can apply the word 'routine' instead, if you'd prefer, but I love the notion of rhythm over routine.

Routine is rigid and inflexible and makes you feel that a set sequence of events needs to happen precisely or the exercise is a failure.

Rhythm, however, is a much friendlier notion. It speaks of order and understanding and flexibility and movement and fluidity.

Even just the sound of the word is friendlier. Rhythm.

Rhythm moves you. You want to dance to rhythm, find your groove, let go a little, enjoy the moment and see where it takes you.

Routine? Not so much.

You need to march to routine. It's a steady metronome keeping time. And if you sway, if you linger, if you move out of order or don't complete a step, you fail. You're out of time. You're lagging behind.

Rhythm allows change and flexibility for the different seasons in life. Which is why I love the approach of rhythm so much more than routine and why I encourage you to spend some time working through the next two exercises to establish morning and evening rhythms that work for you and support the life you want to live.

6

Morning rhythm

Having a rhythm to your mornings means you know what you need to do and how it needs to unfold. It takes the head work out of your morning, so even if you're not an energetic person first thing, you will still be productive. A positive morning rhythm:

1. works for you

2. gives you enough time to get things done

3. takes into account other people's needs

4. has some wiggle room.

And once it's established, you will feel:

- calmer

- more clear-headed

- more prepared

- less likely to lose your temper or chastise yourself

- more inclined to eat breakfast

- more likely to take a brief moment to practise mindfulness.

Instead of starting your day
by responding to the stimulus around you,
you're proactively creating the day
you want to have. When you wake up and
do the most essential things first, you get
a good start to your day. Your mind is
better focused on the rest of your day's
tasks. And you'll do a better job taking
care of the people you love most.

TSH OXENREIDER

Morning rhythm

 30 MINUTES (ONCE)

This exercise is about asking yourself questions, looking at what needs to happen, what you'd like to happen and what works best for you and your family.

You'll need around 30 minutes for this one, but the good news is once you've done the work it doesn't need to be done repeatedly.

Note: For the purpose of this exercise, the 'morning' is up until the point where you and everyone under your roof is dressed and ready to leave the house, whether you actually do or not.

1. SELF-REFLECTION

Start by asking yourself:

- What do my mornings feel like now?

- How do I want my mornings to feel?

- What do I need to get done in the mornings?

- What do I want to get done in the mornings?

2. IDENTIFY YOUR NEEDS AND WANTS

Grab a sheet of paper and a pen. Draw up three columns and label them:

1. Need to happen

2. Want to happen

3. Sequence and time.

In the first column, list all the tasks that need to happen in the morning – things that are non-negotiable for you and your family.

Include anything that applies from the list below, and add any other essentials specific to your life:

- Get up at …

- Make the bed

- Wake the kids

- Shower

- Eat breakfast

- Tidy kitchen

- Pack/run dishwasher

- Get dressed

- Dress kids

- Brush teeth, hair, etc.

- Clear dining table

- Make kids' beds

- Run a load of laundry

- Prepare lunches

- Prepare snacks

- Tidy living areas

- Pick up clothes

- Out the door for work / activities / school at ...

In the second column, note down all the tasks you would like your morning to include – things that may not be essential, but which make your start a more positive one.

Think about what will get your day underway in an uplifting, energetic or beneficial way – something for you, in other words. For example, you may not need to meditate, but you know your day benefits if you do.

3. DECIDE WHAT TO INCLUDE

Now look at the two columns and circle the tasks you want to include in your morning rhythm.

Ensure you include at least one item from the second column. Including self-care in your mornings – even just a small act – is so important for starting the day feeling positive. It means you're far more likely to be happier, kinder and gentler on yourself and others as you move through your morning.

4. ESTIMATE THE TIME NEEDED

Now that you've established what you would like to happen in the mornings, you need to consider time: both the time these circled tasks take, and the time you have available. In the third column, note down approximate times for each task and add up the total amount of time you'll need for your selected morning tasks.

Always round up: add an extra ten minutes to

deal with spills, phone calls, sleep-ins or, if you're really lucky, sleepy morning sex.

If you leave the house for work or other regular commitments, what time do you need to be out the door by?

What time do you currently wake up?

Add your wake-up time to the amount of time your rhythm takes and see how they work together.

If your new rhythm and your current wake-up time work together, fantastic. If not, you need to decide whether to take some tasks away from your morning or get up earlier.

Can any tasks be done the night before to free up a little time in the morning? Perhaps you could make lunches, pack your bag or run a load of laundry in the evening instead?

Also make sure your expectations are not too high. You can only do so much in a given amount of time, and while creating an intentional rhythm for your morning helps maximise that time, it's not a miracle solution that will give you four hours where there used to be just one.

Tweak and shuffle this list and your wake-up time until they fit together nicely, and remember: there is no right or wrong answer – this is about what works for you, your life and your family.

5. FORMALISING IT

Writing everything down may seem rigid at first. But getting it on paper means you are far more likely to commit to your new morning rhythm – even subconsciously.

For the first week or two, perhaps stick your list to the fridge or noticeboard to offer a visual reminder of the rhythm you're creating. You will find it becomes second nature in no time.

You are not locked into this rhythm – you can and should make changes to it as needed, or if it becomes clear that it's no longer working for you. Remember: it's all about making things simpler for you, your life and your family.

MY MORNING RHYTHM

This is my general rhythm for most mornings.

Some days are more challenging than others, but when tasks flow naturally from one to the next, getting through the peak times of the morning feels like less of a chore and I'm definitely able to get through a lot more each day than if I were to just wing it.

The beauty of this rhythm is that if certain things don't happen (I don't get the laundry on, for example) things don't fall apart: I'll just do it later. Similarly, if I don't get time in my office, I know I've either chosen more sleep (a valid choice some mornings!) or the kids have needed me and I'll have the same time available to me tomorrow. It's about being organised enough – but also knowing when to let go.

- Early rise

- Shower and dress

- Meditate (always) and yoga (sometimes)

- Make a cup of tea

- Straight to the office to write

- Work on current writing project

- Stretches when I feel my mind wander

- Kids wake up, my husband gets them breakfast or we eat together

- Make bed

- Clear dining table

- Tidy kitchen

- Put a load of washing on

- Kids do their chores, get dressed, brush teeth, etc

- Do a regular chore, such as cleaning kitchen, changing linen, sweeping floors

- Hang washing

- Out the door for school drop-off.

This rhythm unfolds so naturally now that I don't need to check in with a sequence of tasks or tick items off a list each morning. It's been crafted over time (and changed as needed) to fit neatly in our current life. This is the goal: a rhythm that you don't need to pay attention to, one that just flows. But it will take some time to get there, so I encourage you to stick with the process for a few weeks and makes tweaks and changes as needed, slowly coming to understand what works best for you.

For fast acting relief, try slowing down.

LILY TOMLIN

7

Evening rhythm

Having already established why rhythm makes more sense than routine, we can dive straight into why you should take the time to establish an evening rhythm.

The benefits of an evening rhythm are:

- You have more flexibility to your evening, meaning you can make allowances easily for days that don't fit the normal flow of events.

- You have the benefit of knowing what needs to be done, and everyone else in the home benefits from that familiarity too.

- You can settle gently into the evening – it reduces stress significantly when everyone understands what the evening brings.

- You can prepare yourself for rest. Coming in to the evening with the end in mind (the end being good rest) means you're more likely to get to bed at an appropriate time and with less on your mind.

- You can sleep calmly, knowing you're prepared for the next day – your home is tidy, you know what needs to happen in the morning: you are ready.

Having an evening rhythm saves you time and energy. You can put that time and energy into other things, such as relaxing, pursuing a hobby or spending time with your partner or kids.

Like the morning rhythm exercise in the last chapter, there is some work to be done here. It takes time to list out your tasks and establish a well-considered, helpful rhythm.

But, unlike the morning rhythm, this is a much more flexible approach. You won't need to leave home on time or catch a bus or a train, so there is more space for life to unfold.

EXERCISE

Evening rhythm

 30 MINUTES (ONCE)

Note: For the purpose of this exercise, 'evening' is from dinner onwards.

1. SELF-REFLECTION

Before you begin, ask yourself:

- What do my evenings feel like now?

- How do I want my evenings to feel?

- What do I need to get done in the evenings?

- What do I want to get done in the evenings?

- What can I do in the evening that will help my mornings flow better?

This step of formally reflecting is important. The aim is to help clarify what your priorities are and what needs to happen. Then you can adopt the right evening rhythm for you, adapt it to suit your particular circumstances, implement it and then forget about it. You want it to work so easily in your life that you don't have to focus on it at all.

2. IDENTIFY YOUR NEEDS AND WANTS

Grab a sheet of paper and a pen. Draw up three columns and label them:

1. Need to happen

2. Want to happen

3. Sequence.

In the first column, list all the tasks that need to

happen in the evening – things that are non-negotiable for you and your family.

Include anything that applies from the list below, and add any other essentials specific to your life:

- Clear dining table

- Tidy kitchen

- Pack and run dishwasher / wash dishes

- Give the kids a bath

- Story time

- Put the kids to bed

- Tidy the house

- Shower

- Relax – TV, computer

- Relax – reading, writing

- Pre-bed rituals – tea, bath

- Go to bed at …

In the second column, note down all the tasks you would like your evening to include – things that may not be essential, but which have a positive input.

Think about what will help you prepare for tomorrow and wind down from today – this is the perfect place to include some of the rituals we've already discussed, as well as some of those tasks you identified in your morning rhythm exercise that will help make mornings easier.

Include anything that applies from the list below, and add anything else that is relevant for you.

- Lay out gym clothes / outfit for the morning

- Pack bags

- Make lunches

- Prepare tomorrow's snacks or dinner

- Brain dump

- Three things list

- Gratitude journal

- Screen-free (unplugging) time

- Meditation.

3. DECIDE WHAT TO INCLUDE
IN YOUR RHYTHM

Now look at the two columns and decide which of these tasks should be in your regular evening rhythm.

Circle each task you'd like to include. While most items will come from the first column, ensure you include at least one item from the second. It's important to include self-care rituals in your evening rhythm, as it allows you to end the day with kindness, regardless of how it unfolded.

4. ESTABLISH THE RHYTHM

Once you have decided what your evenings will include, it's time to establish the rhythm.

Ask yourself:

- Which of these tasks is best to do first?

- Which will help finish my day on a positive note?

- Which helps things run more smoothly tomorrow morning?

- Which tasks should be grouped together? (Making dinner, tidying the kitchen and running the dishwasher combine well, for example.)

Work through the list, writing the rough sequence in the third column.

Keep in mind that every day is different, so – again – this sequence is fluid. You can adjust it to your needs. But the more logical and comfortable it is, the more likely you are to stick with it.

If you think you need a visual reminder, by all means stick this list to the fridge or noticeboard for a week or two. It will help to shape your evenings as you get used to the rhythm, but you will find that soon enough you won't need the reminder at all.

MY EVENING RHYTHM

No two evenings are the same for me – some evenings I go to yoga or the gym, for example, but evenings are undoubtedly more comfortable when a well-established rhythm is allowed to unfold, rather than jamming everything in to a set schedule. This is how my evening rhythm usually looks:

- Prepare dinner

- Eat dinner together

- Kids play (usually outside as we don't really do screen time during the week)

- Tidy the kitchen

- Clear dining table

- Pack and run dishwasher

- Tidy up with kids' help

- Bathe/shower kids

- Get kids dressed and ready for bed

- Story time

- Brush teeth

- Bed – story, song

- Shower

- Plan next day – brain dump, three things, gratitude

- Pack bag if heading out early

- Relax – chat, TV, read

- Screen-free time and pre-bed rituals – tea

- Bed – reading, loving, canoodling and general bed-related shenanigans.

PART THREE

CHECKING IN

Adopting some or (ideally) all of these rituals and rhythms into your busy life will undoubtedly help bring comfort and simplicity to your days.

Remember though: it's not designed to be restrictive. The idea is to simplify life, not add more pressure. If at any time these rituals or rhythms are making you feel:

- stressed

- guilty

- overwhelmed

- less flexible

- less comfortable

- less productive

then you need to promise me you will do one thing:

STOP

8

The un-ritual of tilting

None of the rituals or rhythms we've looked at so far will help if they add to the stress and complication of your daily life. That would make them the antithesis of simplicity.

So, while the advice in this chapter may seem to fly in the face of everything I've said to this point, trust that when you put it into practice it really will make sense.

THE FINAL STEP: TILTING

More a mindset than a ritual, tilting is the opposite of balance. A 2009 study by Marcus Birmingham asked the question 'What are happy women doing differently?' And the response was not – as you might imagine – somehow striking the perfect balance between work, life, health, family, passions and spirituality. Rather than aiming for balance – which the women in the study realised was impossible to achieve, stressful to attempt and boring to live – they 'tilted' towards activities and commitments they liked and found meaningful. Towards the area of life that required their attention in a particular moment, intentionally choosing to be there, present, and then intentionally tilted into another area as needed.

Tilting is about being aware of the changing pressures of life and being flexible, while also rejecting the idea that everything needs to be perfectly balanced every single minute of every day and that anything less is a failure.

BUT WHAT ABOUT BALANCE?

For years we've been sold the idea of work–life balance. And if you look at balance as something you need to achieve every day – keeping the scales evenly weighted between your partner, kids, family, friends, yourself, spirituality, health, keeping the home, work – you will struggle to find real balance and expend so much energy simply on trying to create and maintain it.

Frankly, I think this idea of striking a work–life balance is a complete myth. It's damaging and pressures us to achieve something impossible, where a more fluid approach provides the flexibility required to meet the different needs in our life, as and when it's needed.

Instead of exhausting yourself by trying to achieve balance, learn to tilt. To willingly throw things out of balance. And, importantly, learn to be OK with that.

Actually, we need to learn to embrace it!

Simple living is about finding lightness, joy and presence. That's presumably why you're reading this book – to start living a lighter, more joyful life. The rituals we've looked at over the last seven chapters are all designed to help get you there.

But they will do you no good if you don't learn to shift your mindset from one of balance to something more flexible.

- Some days you are extra busy at work – tilt towards simple meals, light home duties and simple rhythms.

- Some days your kids are happy to play independently – tilt towards catching up on tasks around the house.

- Some days you need to recharge – tilt towards being kind to yourself and letting go of the things that don't help with that.

- Some days your kids are sick, or needy, or plain grumpy, meaning you can't get anything done except the very basics – tilt towards supporting the kids and being extra mindful of what's going on for them.

- Some days your partner is under added pressure at work – tilt towards lessening the load on them at home.

- Some days you need to regain order at home – tilt away from social engagements and towards time spent focused on those needs.

Tilting allows us to focus on what's important in the moment, and intentionally choose to put our energies into those areas. The physical act of tilting means we're leaning in to one thing, and leaning out of another. We can't be everything to everyone in every moment, and tilting makes it clear that by saying yes to one thing, we're saying no to another in that moment. And what's more, it's OK to do so.

Conversely, tilting actually helps us to achieve balance over a longer period of time. Instead of battling to find it every day, it's more important to create balance over a month – or a year. If we take a longer view of balance, it's much easier to see if we're living the way we want to be, or what areas we need to focus on more. Plus, we all have bad days and stressful times and it's far more forgiving to take a broader view of balance – chances are, if you're tilting in to the

important things, you'll find you've achieved
that balance over time.

HOW TO TILT

It's not a matter of learning a step-by-step
approach. It's more about keeping the idea of
tilting in the back of your mind.

It's about understanding – and accepting –
the fact that you can not and will not ever achieve
perfect balance.

What's more, you probably wouldn't want to.

Achieving and then maintaining a state of
balanced perfection would be incredibly stressful
and unfulfilling. Instead, understand that your
time is limited and valuable. And you can choose
where to place your energies, depending upon
where they need to be.

Your life is yours.

I can't tell you where your priorities need to
lie. But every once in a while, ask yourself if you
feel balanced:

- this week?

- this month?

- in the past six months?

The answer you feel in your gut will guide you much better than any ideal of perfect daily balance will.

The quality of life is in proportion, always, to the capacity for delight. The capacity for delight is the gift of paying attention.

JULIA CAMERON

9

Noticing

So much of simple living is in the art of noticing. Stopping long enough to attend to the beauties – both large and tiny – that surround us. In fact, if I had to sum this book up in one idea it would be this: become a noticer. Slow down and pay attention.

To pay attention is to give of yourself. There is a cost involved in paying attention. But there is also a cost involved in not paying attention, and that cost is far steeper. Pay attention to:

• what you do and how it feels

• what you consume

- the things you need to do

- how you feel as you do them

- the spaces in between

- your thoughts and feelings

- beauty

- your time and energy

- where you spend it.

Pay attention to what the world is trying to show you.

10

Go, enjoy life!

I hope you're still feeling motivated to simplify your daily life using these rituals and rhythms, because now you get to start using them to create your simpler, happier, lighter life.

Just like any changes in life, you will need to adjust your rhythms and rituals over time. As your life moves and shifts, you will find your needs move and shift with it.

Whenever you feel life becoming unbalanced or you find yourself feeling overwhelmed again, take that as a cue to revisit the exercises in *Destination Simple*. You may just need to remind yourself of the work you've laid out, or you may find that life has changed enough for you to reassess what still works and what no longer does.

I truly think anyone who reads this book can benefit from the rituals and rhythms I describe in these pages. Even if you only include one of these rituals in your day, I'm confident it will improve life for you. I'm so passionate, though, about the benefits of living a simpler life, that I would love to see you put them all in to practice. That's where the biggest benefits lie.

Give yourself one or two weeks to try these rituals in your everyday life.

Once that time has passed, look at your life, your heart and your head, and ask yourself: Do I feel more prepared for my days, more even-handed, happier, more content, more organised, more in control?

In the meantime, go enjoy life. That's what all this work is about – creating a slower, simpler life that gives you the time and space for more of what you enjoy.

And thank you for taking the time to read this little book.

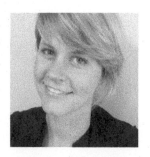

Brooke McAlary and her husband, Ben, produce and host The Slow Home Podcast, an iTunes #1 Health program, where they discuss slow living in all its different forms.

You can learn more about Brooke and her simple living mission at slowyourhome.com.